CUTS AND BURNS

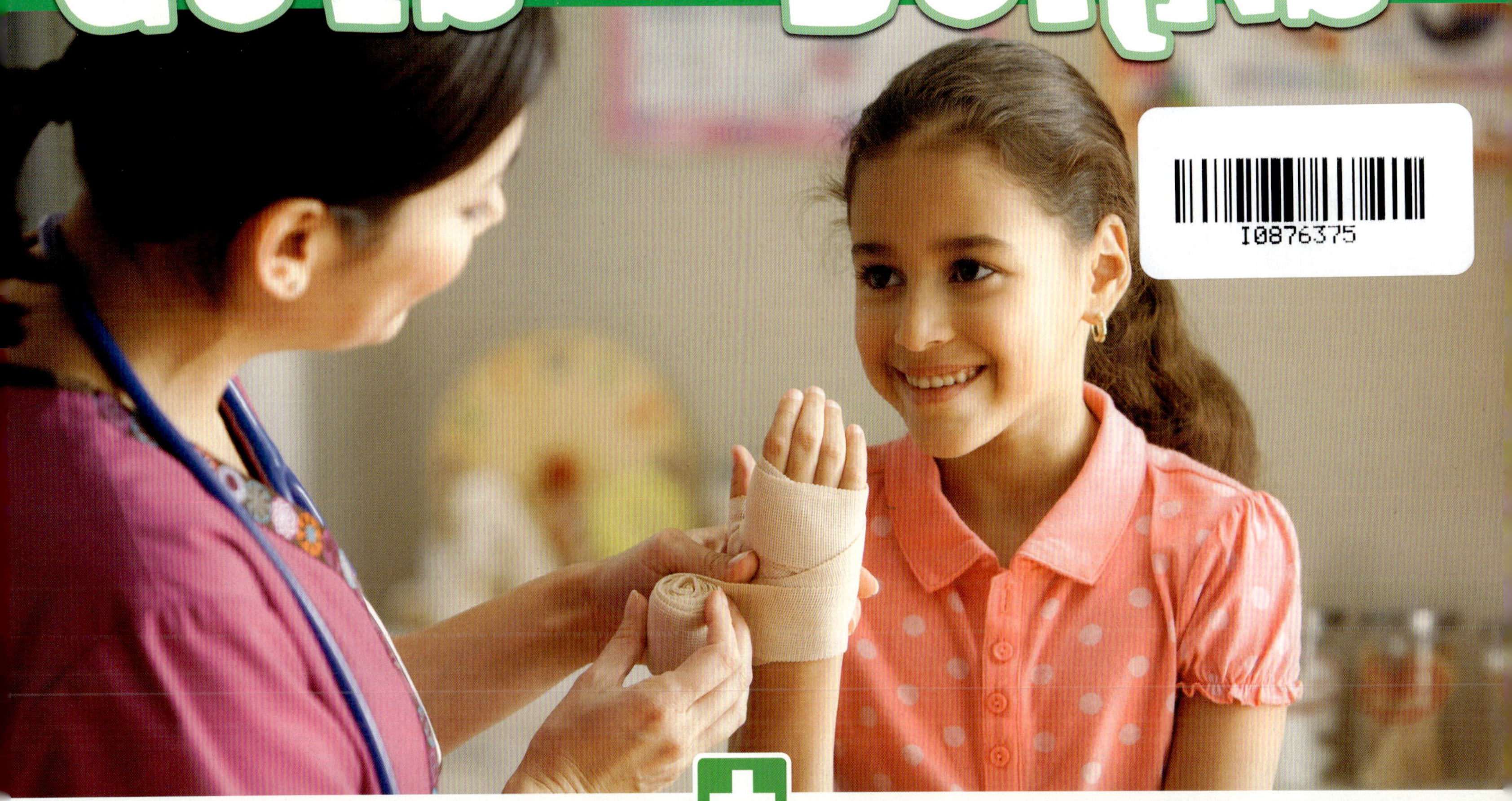

IN CASE OF EMERGENCY

Jacqueline S. Cotton
and Ryan Smith

AV2
www.av2books.com

Step 1
Go to www.av2books.com

Step 2
Enter this unique code
CDLNRIDZY

Step 3
Explore your interactive eBook!

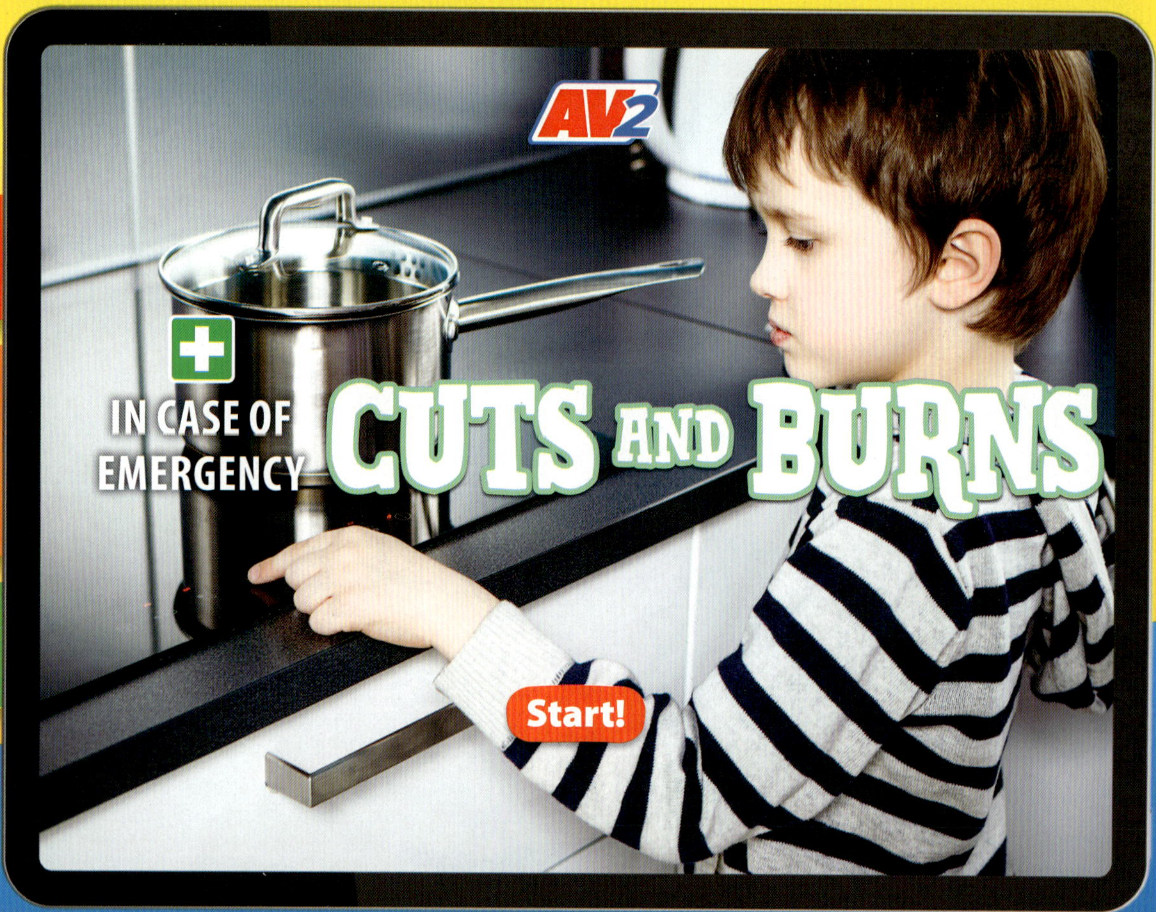

AV2 is optimized for use on any device

Your interactive eBook comes with...

Audio
Listen to the entire book read aloud

Videos
Watch informative video clips

Weblinks
Gain additional information for research

Try This!
Complete activities and hands-on experiments

Key Words
Study vocabulary, and complete a matching word activity

Quizzes
Test your knowledge

Slideshows
View images and captions

View new titles and product videos at www.av2books.com

IN CASE OF EMERGENCY

CUTS AND BURNS

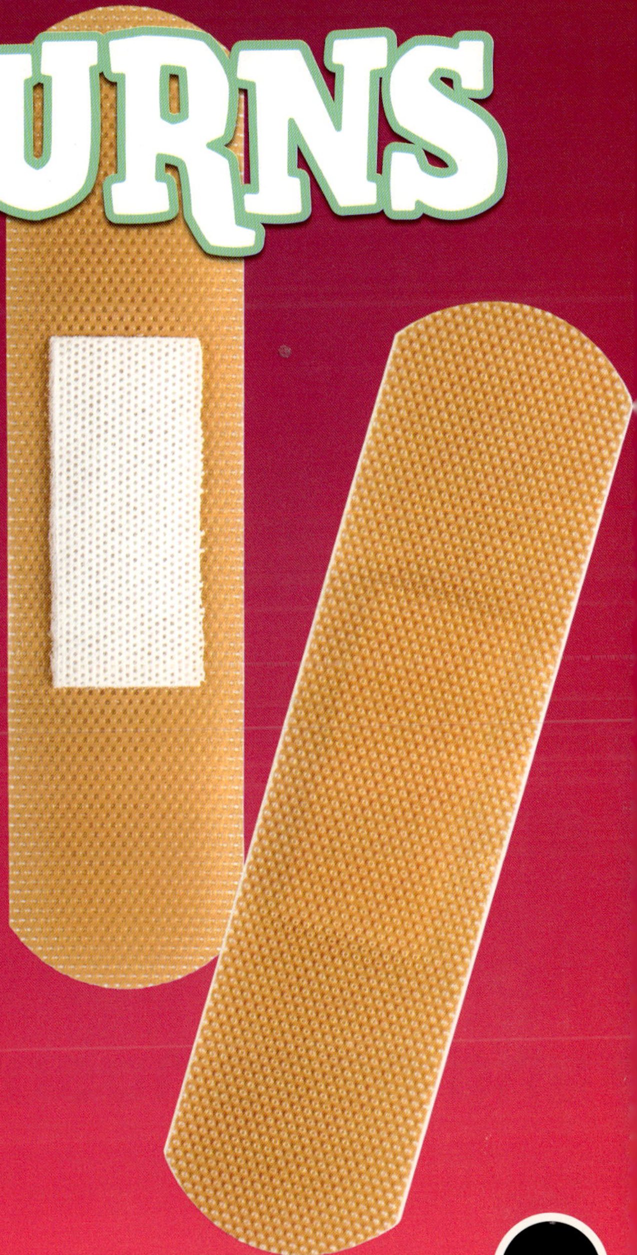

Contents

Cuts and Burns

Cuts and burns are common injuries.

Many of these injuries are small and can be treated at home.

Some are more serious and need hospital treatment.

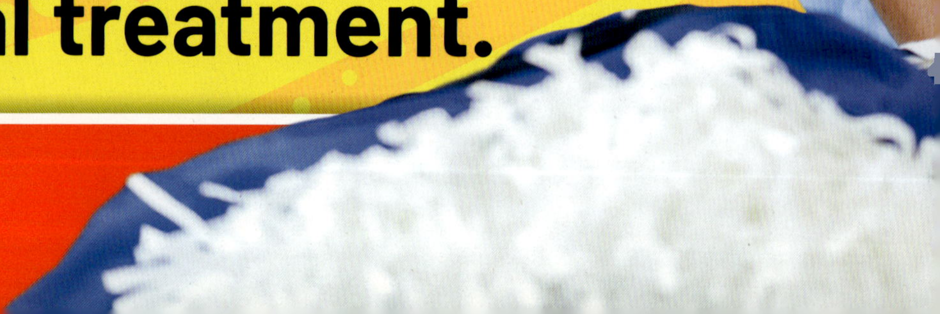

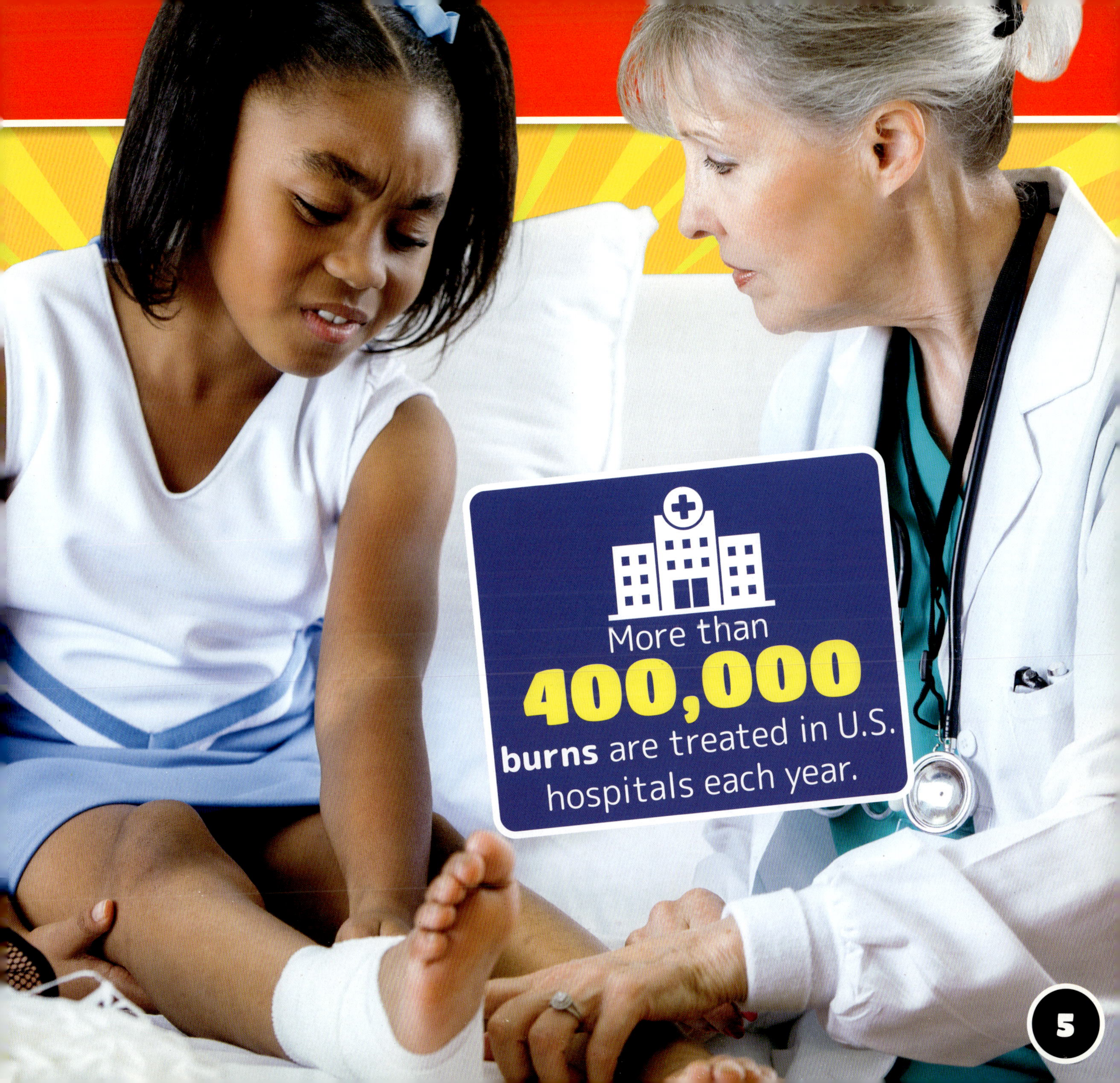

More than

400,000

burns are treated in U.S. hospitals each year.

Signs and Symptoms

A person gets a cut when something sharp breaks his or her skin. Cuts may start to bleed.

If a person touches something that is very hot, he or she might get burned. A burn will turn skin red and make it blister.

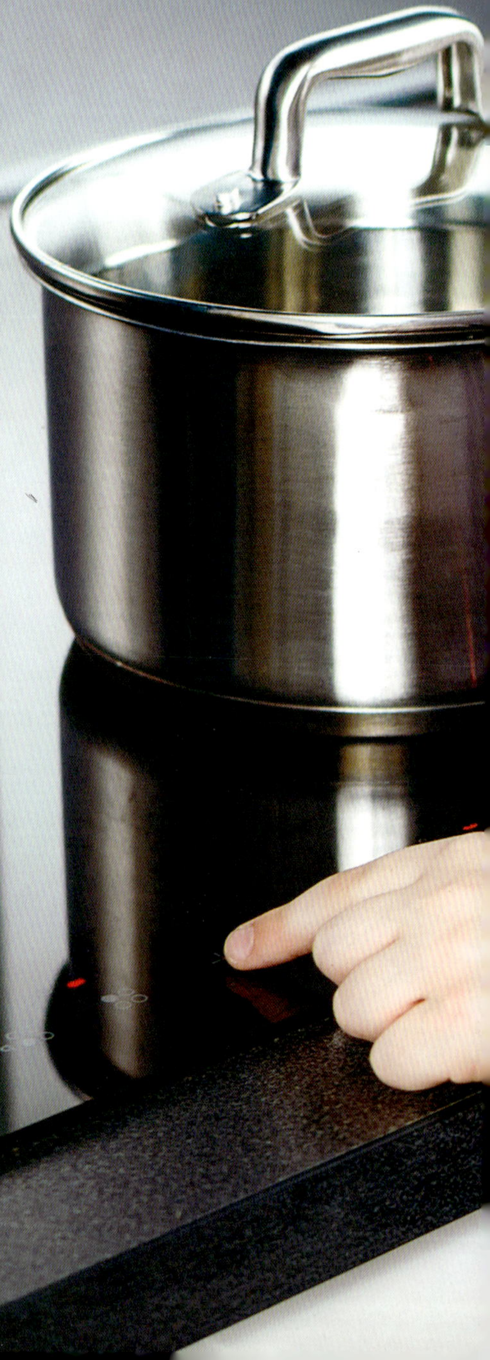

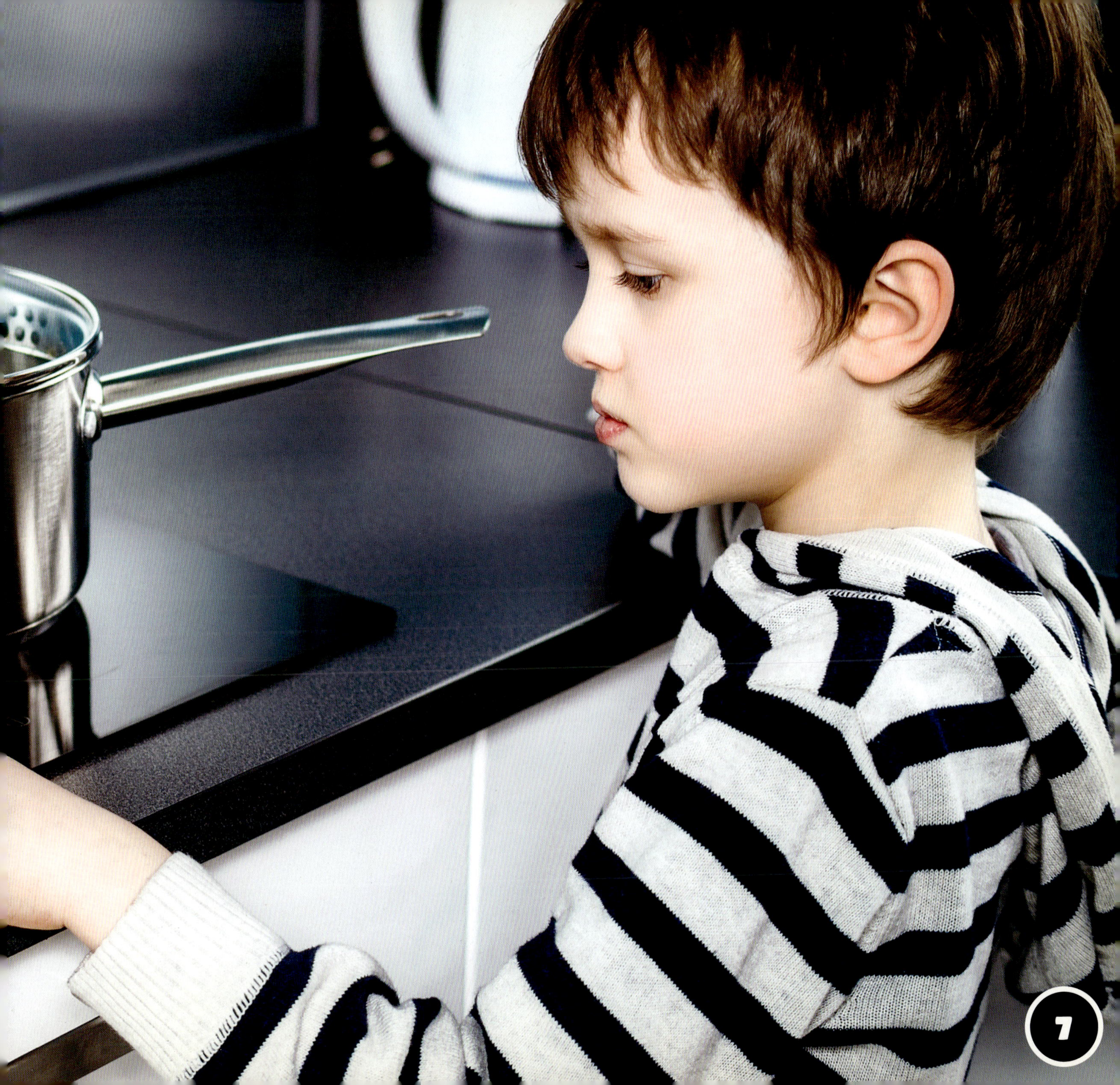

Stay Calm

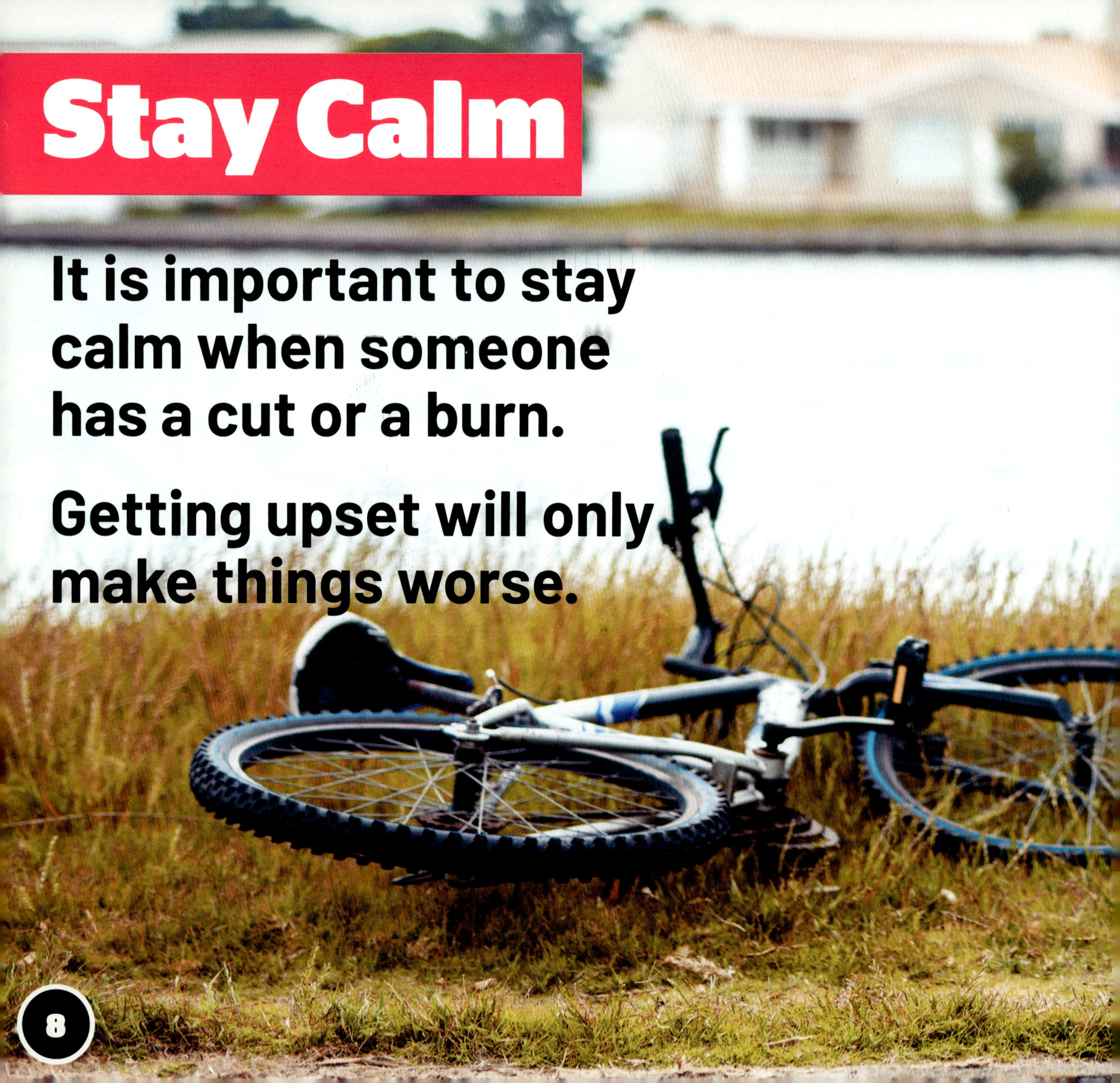

It is important to stay calm when someone has a cut or a burn.

Getting upset will only make things worse.

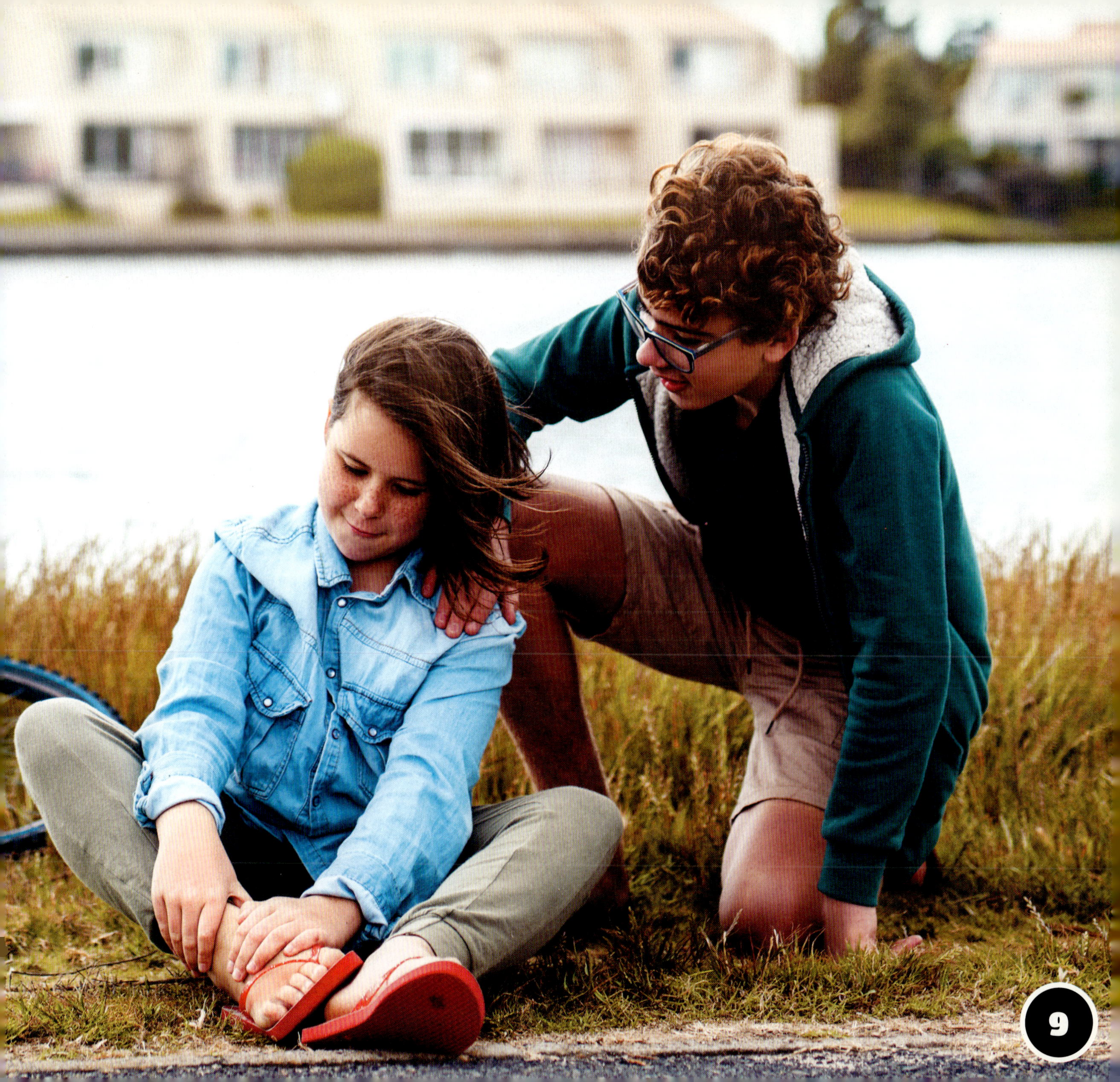

Call 9-1-1

Call 9-1-1 if a cut or a burn is really bad.

The 9-1-1 operator will need to know your name, where you are, and what the emergency is.

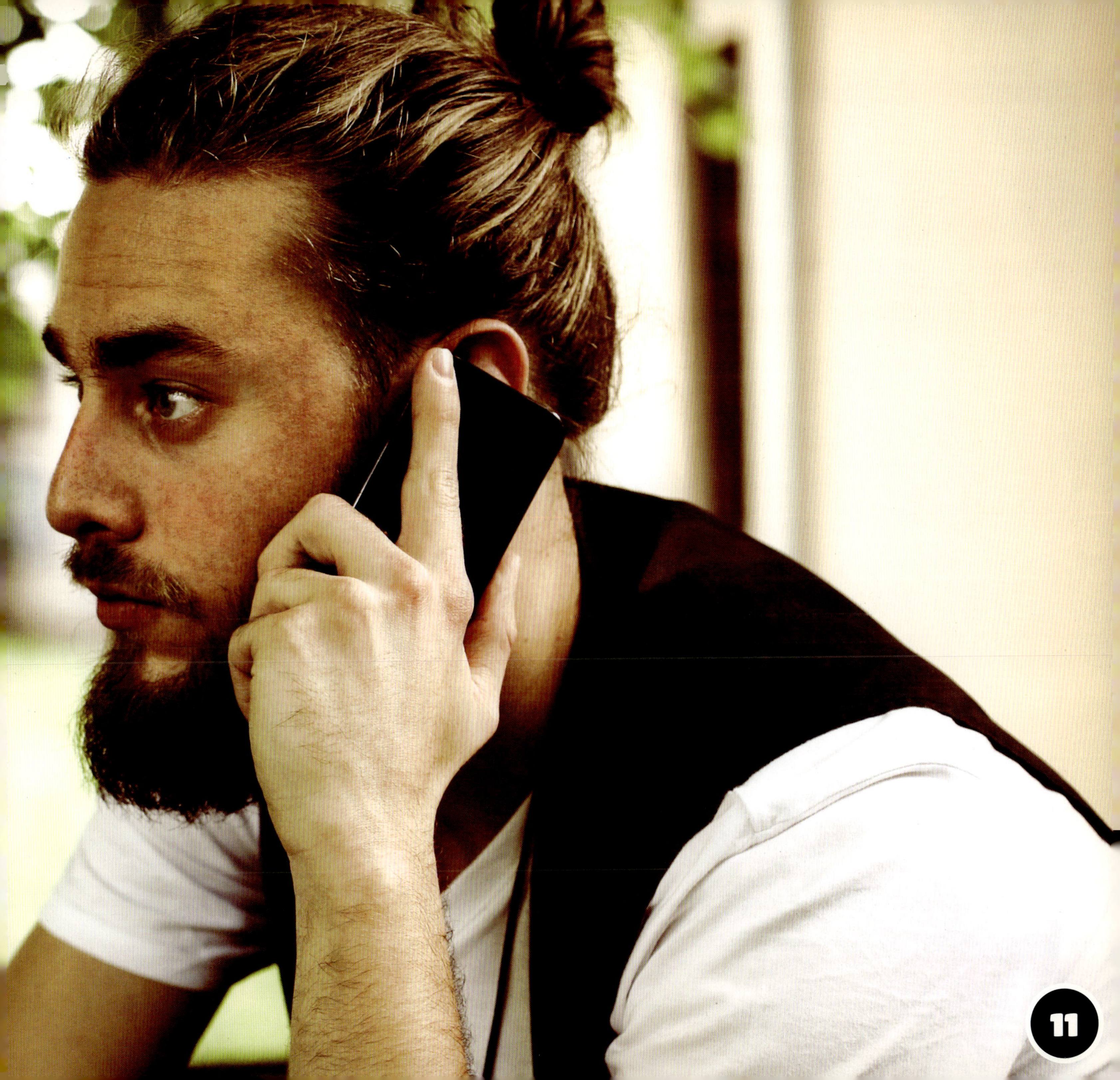

Get a First Aid Kit

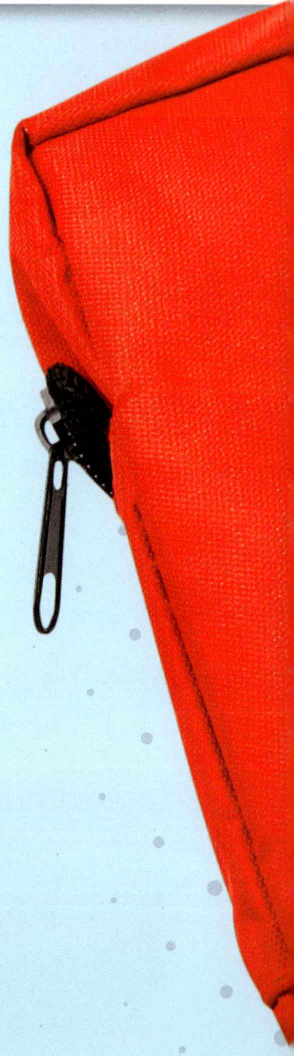

A first aid kit can help with a cut or a burn.

It has supplies for treating injuries.

A first aid kit may be kept in the school office.

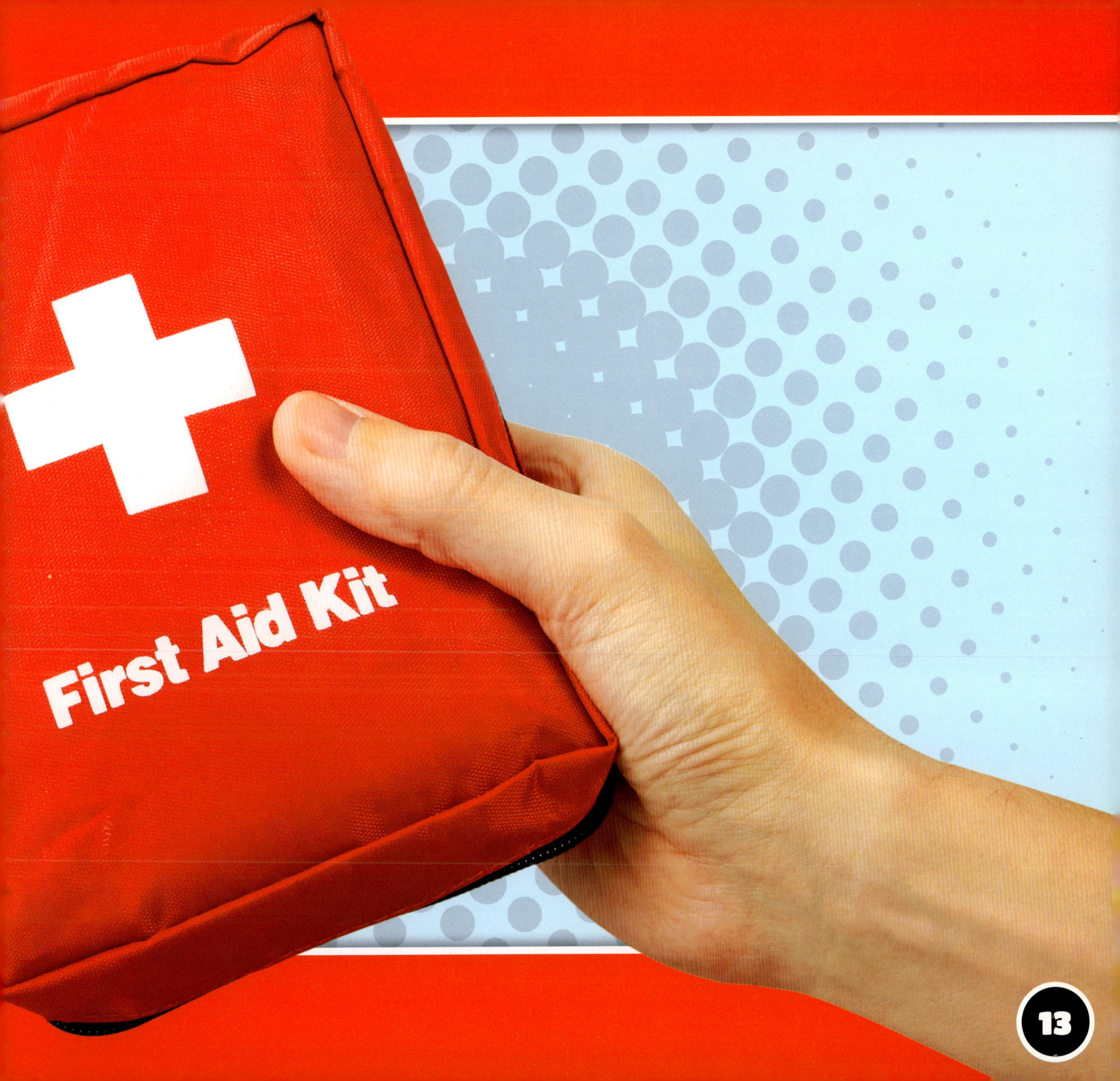
First Aid Kit

Wash with Water

Wash cuts with running water to get rid of dirt and germs.

If someone has a burn, run cool water over the injury.

This will cool it down.

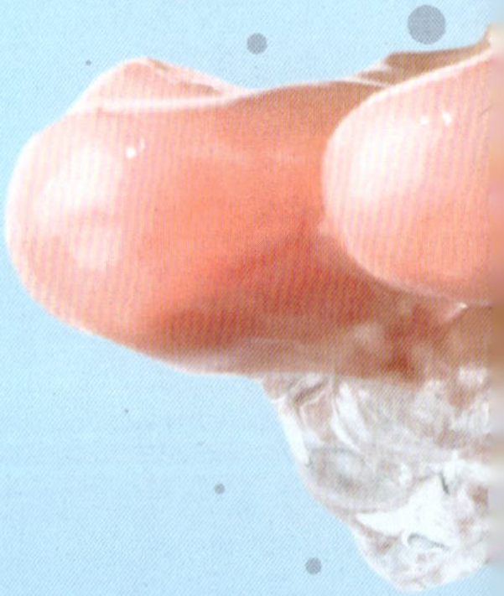

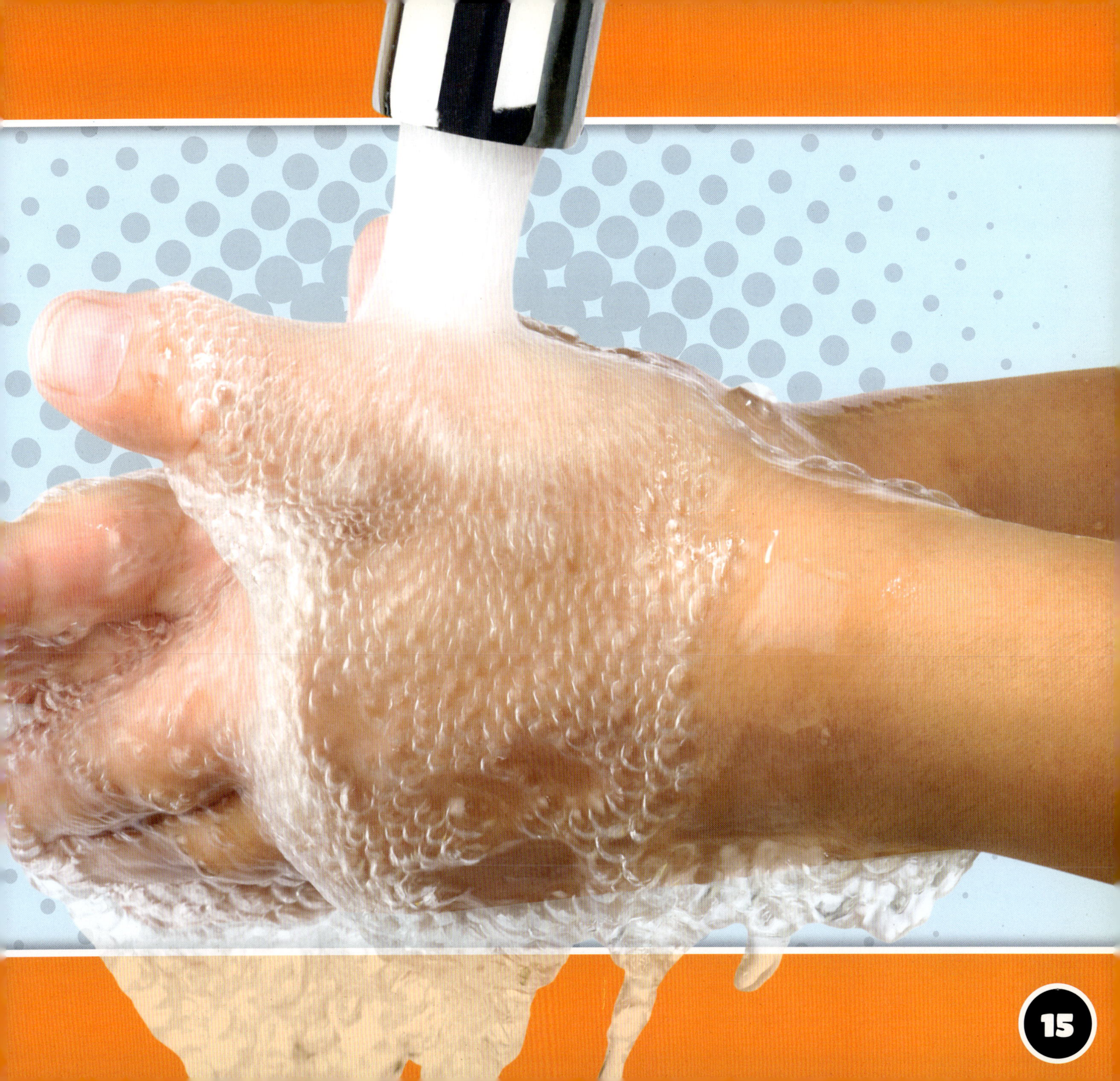

Cover the Cut or Burn

Cover a cut or burn with a clean bandage or a soft cloth.

This will help keep germs and dirt out of the cut or burn.

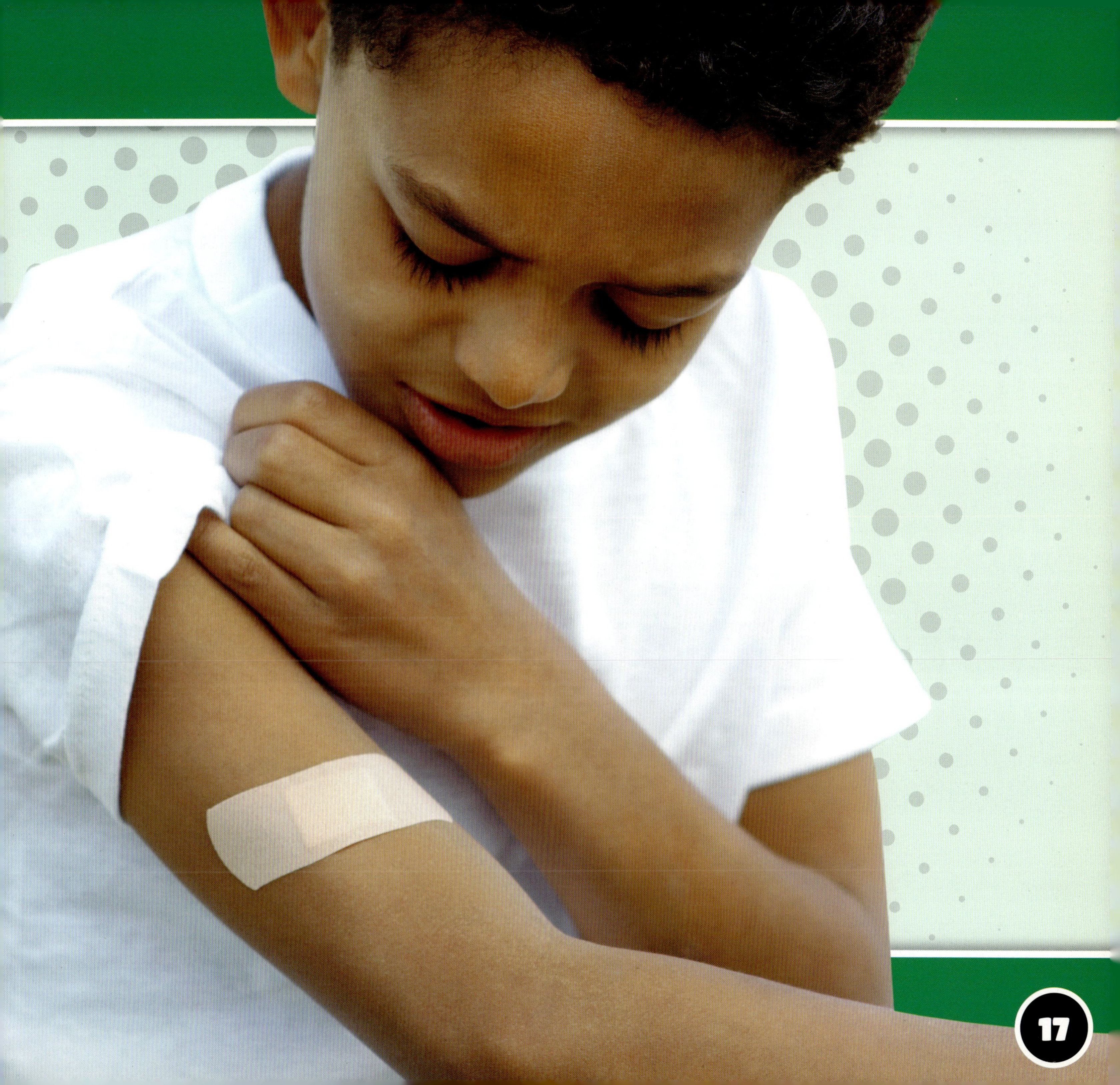

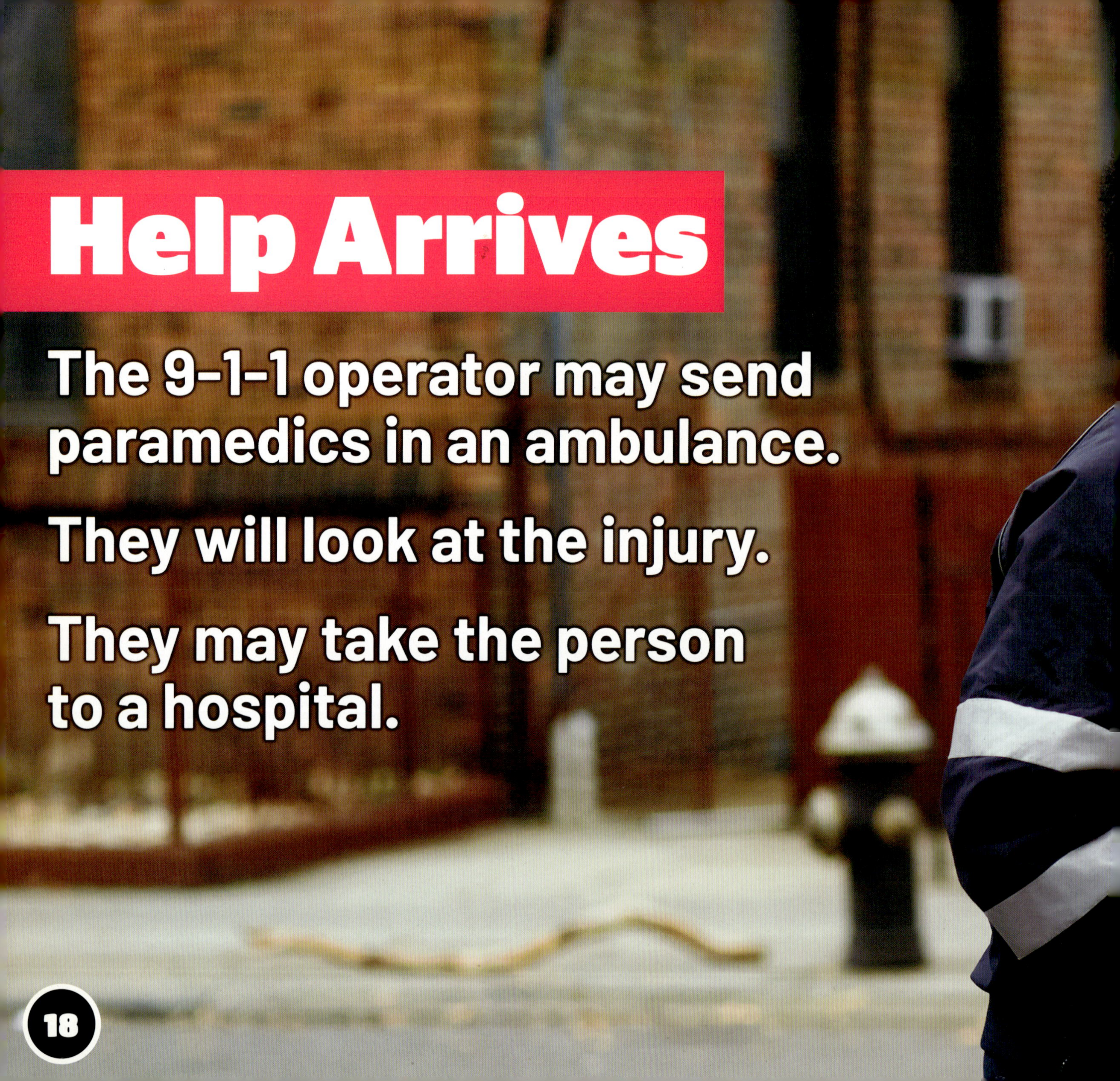

Help Arrives

The 9-1-1 operator may send paramedics in an ambulance.

They will look at the injury.

They may take the person to a hospital.

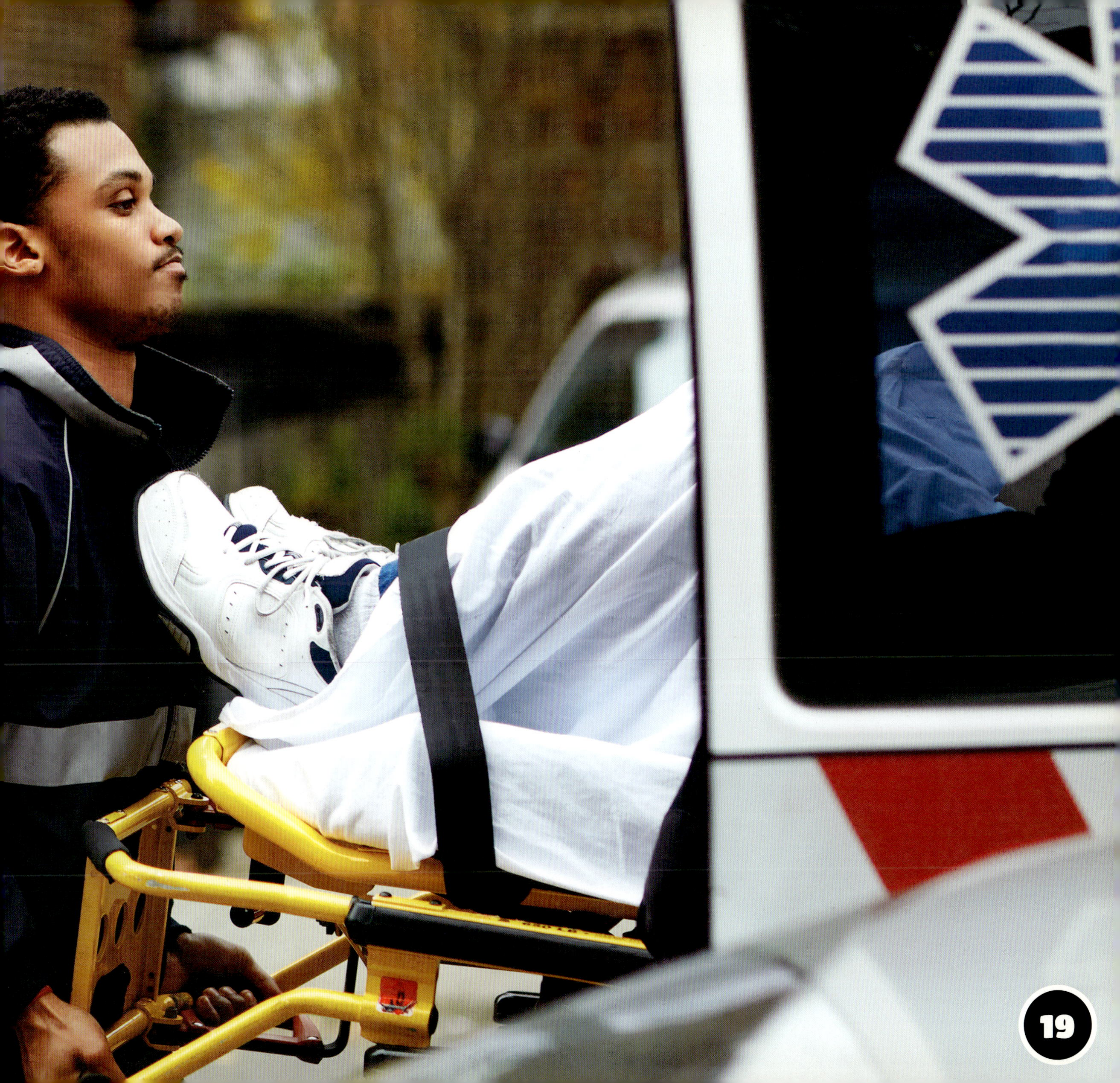

Preventative Measures

People should be careful when they handle sharp or hot things.

Following safety rules helps to prevent cuts and burns.

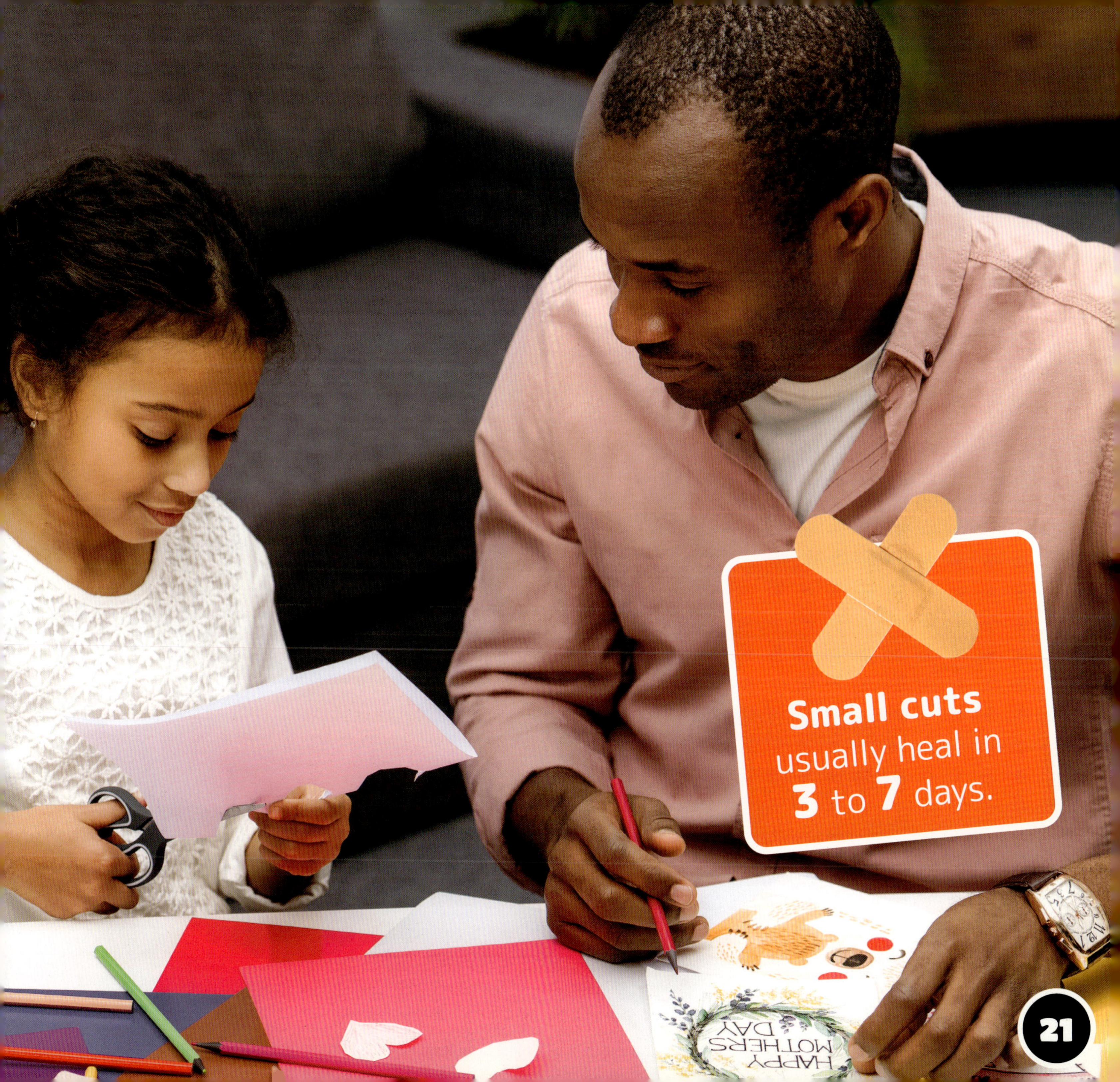

Small cuts usually heal in **3** to **7** days.

EMERGENCY PROCEDURES

These pages provide detailed information that expands on the emergency found in the book. They are intended to be used by adults as a learning support to help young readers understand the correct responses to each emergency featured in the *In Case of Emergency* series.

Pages 4–5

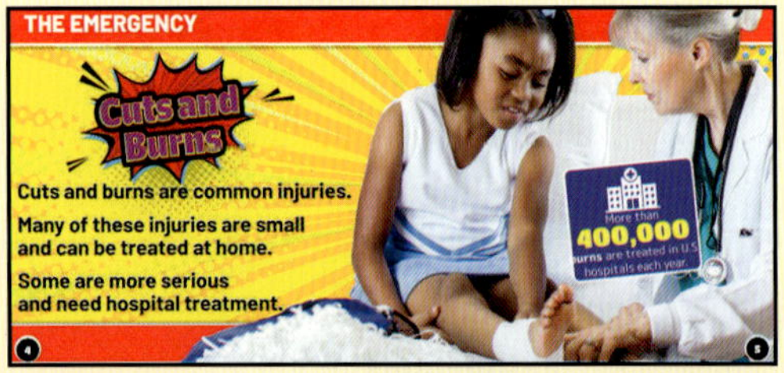

Cuts and burns are common injuries. Some cuts and burns are minor, but others are medical emergencies. Cuts are caused by something sharp or abrasive breaking the skin. A burn is caused by excessive heat being applied to the skin. A person will instinctively react to either of these injuries.

Pages 6–7

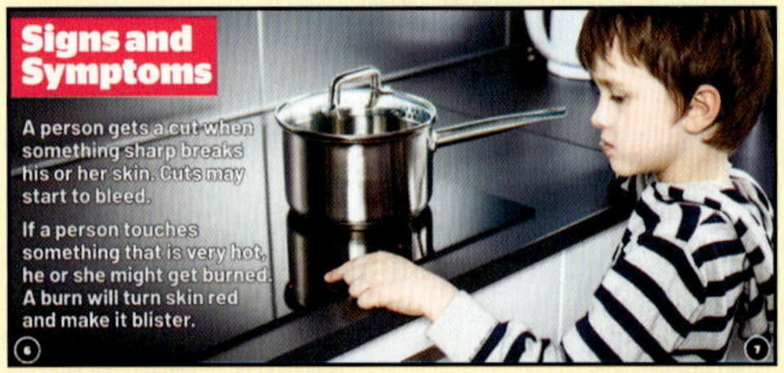

A person gets a cut when something sharp breaks his or her skin. Cuts will bleed as the body attempts to flush and clot the wound. More severe cuts may reveal the muscle and bone beneath the skin. A burn causes the affected area to turn red and blister. Serious burns will scorch the skin and burn the deeper tissues beneath it.

Pages 8–9

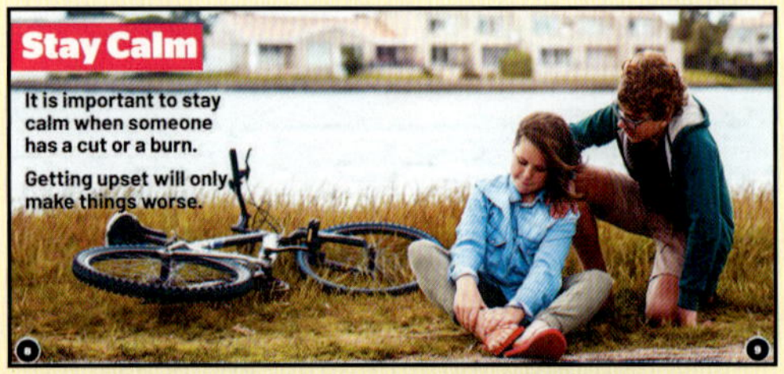

It is important to stay calm when someone has a cut or a burn. It is especially important for the injured person to remain calm. Panicking can make a cut bleed faster, agitate a burn, or send the injured person into shock. If you are the person assisting someone with a cut or a burn, stay calm. This will help prevent mistakes from being made while treating the injuries. It will also help the injured person stay calm.

Pages 10–11

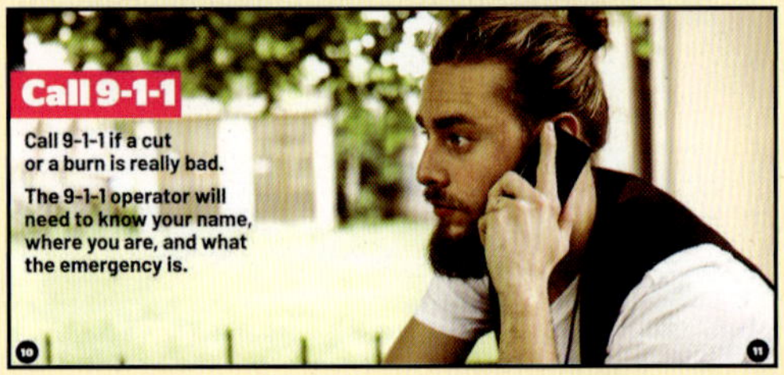

Call 9-1-1 if a cut or a burn is really bad. A call to 9-1-1 should only be placed in emergency situations. Depending on the severity of a cut or burn, calling 9-1-1 may be necessary. The injury should be assessed to determine if it is a major or minor injury. Major injuries, such as deep cuts or large burns, are more serious and need immediate professional medical care. Minor injuries can usually be treated at home.

Pages 12–13

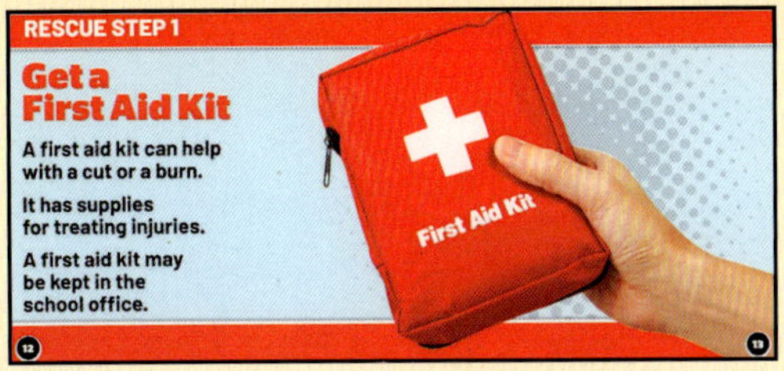

A first aid kit can help with a cut or a burn. A first aid kit should include gauze, medical tape, bandages, non-latex gloves, ice packs, wipes, hand sanitizers, tweezers, and more. First aid kits should be easy to identify and stored in a common location. Inspecting first aid kits on a regular basis ensures medical supplies are restocked and have not expired. It is important to wash your hands before and after providing first aid. This prevents infections and the spreading of germs. It is also important to wear gloves when administering first aid to avoid transferring bodily fluids.

Pages 14–15

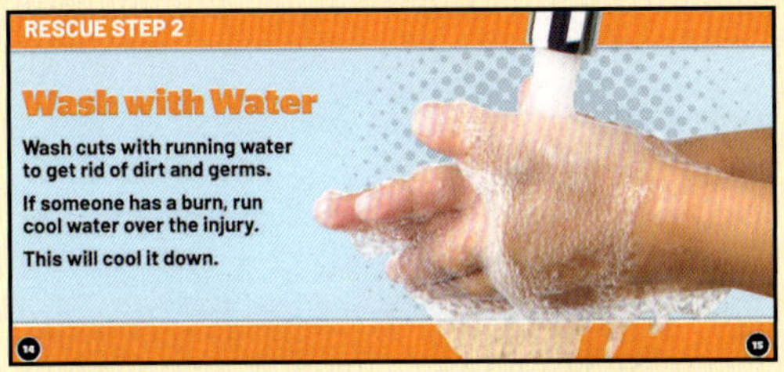

Wash cuts with running water to get rid of dirt and germs. The bleeding must be stopped before a cut can be washed. Use a sterile gauze or soft cloth to apply gentle pressure to the wound. Then, flush out the cut with running water to wash out bacteria and debris. Depending on the severity and location of a burn, it can be treated by running cool water over the wound. This cools down the burned area, relieves pain, and speeds up the healing process.

Pages 16–17

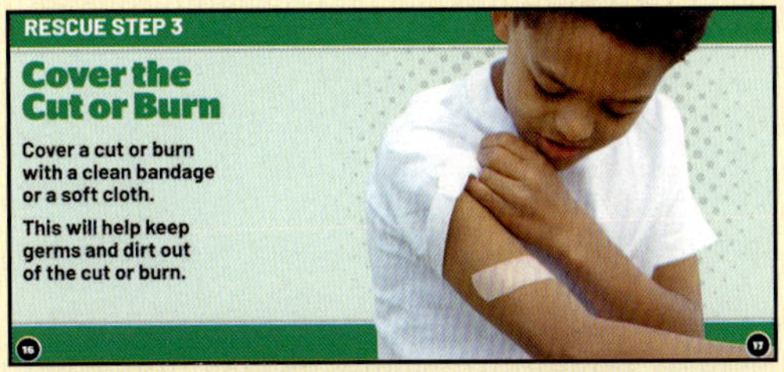

Cover a cut or burn with a clean bandage or a soft cloth. After cleaning a cut, cover it with a sterile bandage or gauze and medical tape. This helps the healing process and prevents infections. Change the bandage if it gets wet or dirty. Like a cut, a burn should be covered. Use a dry, sterile, non-stick bandage or gauze and medical tape to cover the burn. Place the gauze loosely over the burn. Covering the burn helps protect the skin, decreases the risk of infection, and eases the pain.

Pages 18–19

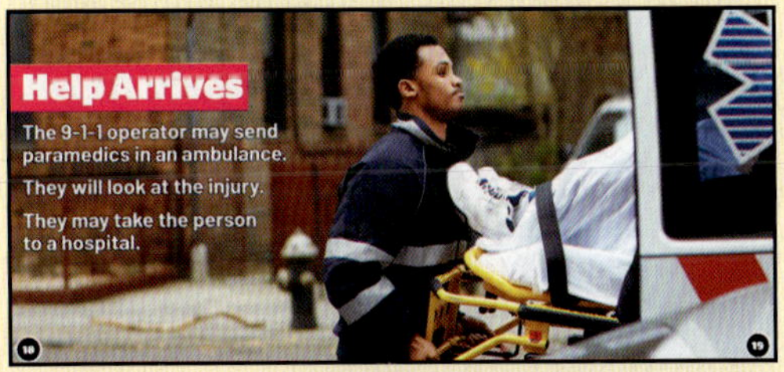

The 9-1-1 operator may send paramedics in an ambulance. Paramedics will assess the injuries and begin to provide the appropriate treatments. They will also monitor the injured person for shock. If the injuries are severe enough, paramedics will take the injured person to a hospital. At the hospital, doctors will be able to stitch up large cuts so they can heal more quickly. Doctors can also begin to treat skin that has been damaged by severe burns.

Pages 20–21

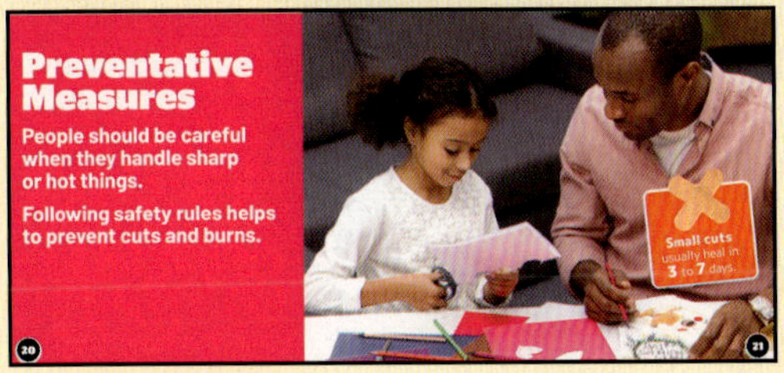

People should be careful when they handle sharp or hot things. Avoid cuts and burns by staying aware of what could harm you. Follow safety rules and make them a habit. The kitchen is a good example of a place where awareness and rules can keep a person from getting a cut or burn. There are many sharp objects and hot surfaces in a kitchen. Listening to adults and being aware of the surroundings will help a person stay safe in the kitchen.

KEY WORDS

Research has shown that as much as 65 percent of all written material published in English is made up of 300 words. These 300 words cannot be taught using pictures or learned by sounding them out. They must be recognized by sight. This book contains 74 common sight words to help young readers improve their reading fluency and comprehension. This book also teaches young readers several important content words, such as proper nouns. These words are paired with pictures to aid in learning and improve understanding.

Page	Sight Words First Appearance
4	and, are, at, be, can, cuts, home, many, more, need, of, small, some, the, these
5	each, in, than, year
6	a, gets, he, her, his, if, important, is, it, make, may, might, or, she, something, start, that, to, turn, very, when, will
8	important, has, only, things
10	call, know, name, really, what, where, you, your
12	first, for, help, one, school, with
14	down, over, run, this, water
16	keep, out
18	an, look, take, they
20	following, people, should
21	days

Page	Content Words First Appearance
4	burns, cuts, emergency, hospital, injuries, treatment
6	person, signs, skin, symptoms
10	operator
12	first aid kit, office, step, supplies
14	dirt, germs
16	bandage, cloth
18	ambulance, paramedics
20	preventative measures, rules

Published by AV2
14 Penn Plaza 9th Floor New York, NY 10122
Website: www.av2books.com

Library of Congress Cataloging-in-Publication Data

Names: Cotton, Jacqueline S., author. | Smith, Ryan, author.
Title: Cuts and burns / Jacqueline S. Cotton, Ryan Smith.
Description: New York, NY : AV2, [2021] | Series: In case of emergency | Audience: Ages 5-9 | Audience: Grades 2-3
Identifiers: LCCN 2020014404 (print) | LCCN 2020014405 (ebook) | ISBN 9781791126643 (library binding) | ISBN 9781791126650 (paperback) | ISBN 9781791126667 | ISBN 9781791126674
Subjects: LCSH: Wounds and injuries--Juvenile literature. | Burns and scalds--Juvenile literature. | Medical emergencies--Juvenile literature.
Classification: LCC RC87 .C765 2021 (print) | LCC RC87 (ebook) | DDC 617.1/1--dc23
LC record available at https://lccn.loc.gov/2020014404
LC ebook record available at https://lccn.loc.gov/2020014405

Printed in Guangzhou, China
1 2 3 4 5 6 7 8 9 0 24 23 22 21 20

052020
100919

Project Coordinator: Ryan Smith
Art Director: Terry Paulhus

The publisher acknowledges Getty Images, iStock, and Shutterstock as its primary image suppliers for this title.